WEIGHT LOSS

Losing Weight The Right Way

A Book on Healthy Weight Loss and Weight Management

PAOLO JOSE DE LUNA

Table of Contents

Paolo Jose De Luna

Introduction

Food is one of the most important basic needs that humans cannot live without. For this reason, we have to look for food to meet our daily nutritional needs. In recent years, humans have found easy ways to obtain food and meet their everyday dietary needs. The modern food industry has also grown tremendously with the introduction of innovative food production methods. As a result, people around the world are able to get delicious foods that didn't exist several years ago. Today's food industry has experienced significant changes making it possible for people to acquire the food they need without waiting for too long. Generally, food is readily available in different forms and is easy to find, unlike before.

One of the key changes that have taken place as a result of the ever-growing food industry is the availability of food in shops. People have established many shops in all parts of the world. Consequently, we can easily find the food we need at the nearest store without having to travel long distances. So, whenever we feel hungry and there is no food in the house, we only need to walk to the local shop and purchase some foodstuffs to satiate our hunger.

Without a doubt, the growing food industry has made food an easy-to-find commodity thanks to incredible innovations around the globe. However, it's important to acknowledge that many people are at a greater risk of gaining weight because of the types of foods we eat every day.

Weight loss has become a key concern for many people around the world. This is happening because of the increasing number of people who are becoming overweight. In fact, many people have gained too much weight to the extent of becoming obese. The truth of the matter is that an overweight or obese person is likely to develop health problems. Some of the common health problems associated with weight gain include heart-related diseases like hypertension, myocardial infarction (MI), and atherosclerosis. Excess body weight can also contribute to the development of health problems such as chronic obstructive pulmonary disease (COPD), diabetes mellitus, and cerebrovascular disease.

You are most likely to be aware of the reasons why many people are concerned about losing weight. There are obvious clues including visiting the gym on a regular basis, restricting oneself to specific diets, avoiding certain types of dishes, and engaging in other practices just to lose some weight. Generally, people are doing everything possible to lose weight or avoid gaining weight. For those looking for ways to lose weight, the truth is that it is not an easy process. It's quite a journey and you must be prepared. You have to invest your time, spend some money, and uphold a certain level of discipline. Above all, you must set goals and work hard so you can achieve the desired results within a specified period of time if possible.

People who want to begin the weight loss process have a wide range of options to choose from including medical methods inspired by science as well as natural methods. Whatever method you choose, you have to keep in mind the possible consequences. If you decide to use scientific methods, you have the option to undergo surgical procedures to drain excess fat from your body. Obviously, surgery is an easy method of removing excess fat from the body, but there are significant consequences including the possibility of developing some serious complications. Surgery will help remove fat beneath the skin surface, but you will struggle with loose skin after the procedure. Fat causes the skin to stretch so you should expect your skin to become saggy if you choose surgery as you weight loss option.

The best way to lose weight is to use a combination of practices that reduce the chances of developing complications and undesired outcomes. These including choosing a healthy diet, doing exercises on a regular basis, and adopting a healthy lifestyle. If you want to lose weight and try to look for help, you'll come across articles, endorsements, and people who promise to offer a shortcut. However, you should always remember that no shortcut method will help you lose body weight overnight.

As mentioned earlier, weight loss is a process that needs a lot of effort and time. Therefore, you can expect to spend a lot of your time, which could be several weeks or months before you start to see the results you expected. The bottom line is that you must work hard if you wish to lose some extra pounds. You'll eventually achieve good results if you stay focused and remain patient throughout the process.

This is the right book if you look forward to losing those unwanted pounds. By reading this book, you'll learn everything you need to know about weight loss. Read on to learn the correct steps you need to take to lose weight the correct way. You definitely want to avoid unhealthy practices and the usual weight loss habits that might be harmful to your health. Many unhealthy weight loss habits and contemporary trends will only make you feel hungrier, weaken your body, and discourage you because they are not effective methods of losing weight. The good news is that this book only focuses on natural methods that will help you lose weight without causing complications or undesirable results.

One of the key determinants of a successful weight loss story is the type of knowledge you have before you start the journey. You must have the right knowledge in addition to being smart. Failure to get the right information means you are likely to waste your resources including your precious time. No one wants to waste money on something that will eventually lead to annoying outcomes and regrets. This book will provide you with the knowledge you need to lose weight using the right methods and without wasting your money and time. Continue reading to find out more. Let's get started!

CHAPTER 1:

Getting Started

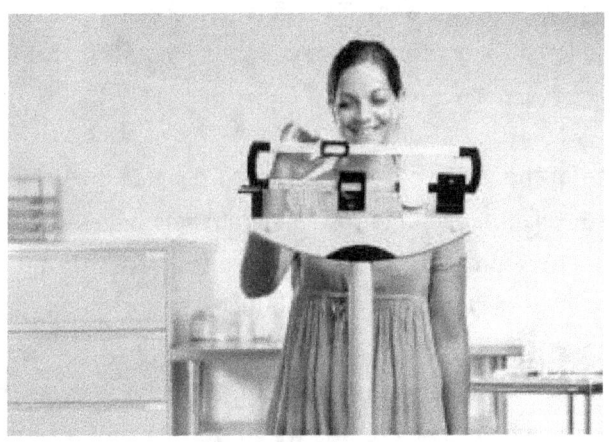

With the increasing number of people who want to lose weight, chances are you've also set a goal to lose a few pounds or maintain your weight. You are not alone because many people have attempted to use weight loss and weight management methods. Nowadays, it's easy to find discussions and talks about how to lose weight and the benefits of weight loss. Such discussions attract a lot of attention because people who have gained unwanted weight or developed obesity are more likely to suffer from health problems such as hypertension and diabetes mellitus. Such people hope to find an effective weight loss solution.

If you've listened to weight loss discussions and tried some supposedly effective methods just to lose those extra pounds or maintain your own body weight, you are probably aware of the fact that weight loss does not happen instantly. Weight is a time-consuming process that demands a lot of work. Therefore, anyone who wants to lose weight should know that it is not a simple task that can be completed overnight.

One of the major problems faced by people who want to lose weight is the urge to give up at some point and stop the entire process. If you allow this to happen, it means you've been working hard for nothing. Many people usually decide to stop if they get no results or insignificant results that do not meet their expectations. Obviously, it is easy for anyone who is trying to lose weight to give up if their diet plan and workout programs fail. Similarly, you are likely to feel wasted after all the mental effort you've invested and the sacrifices you've made just to shave off the extra pounds in your body.

However, if you are really determined to lose those surplus pounds, there is no reason to turn back after all the investments you've made from the start. The weight loss journey has its ups and downs just like any other journey. You need to be resilient, patient, and persistent to achieve your goal. If you realize that you are not making any progress, don't give up. Keep trying and hope for the best because nothing is impossible. Perhaps you've been doing things the wrong way and you need to lose weight the right way.

You've probably heard stories of people who have tried to lose weight and succeeded. They now have good-shaped bodies with the curves everyone wishes to have, but you have not been able to get the same results. Maybe you've read many books about weight loss, watched a lot of weight loss commercials or videos, and done everything possible based on the information you've acquired, but things aren't getting better than they were before. Perhaps you are tired and you are no longer interested, but you should not let your past experiences pull you down. Don't give up because there's always a chance to lose weight as long as you use the right weight loss methods.

There are several factors that make you different from any other person who is trying to lose weight. For this reason, you may not succeed if you rely on other people's weight loss programs. Someone may use a certain regimen and achieve the desired results, but it does not mean that the same regimen will work for you. This means that you could be using the wrong regimen and that's why all your efforts seem to be in vain. So, if the weight loss program you've been using doesn't seem to bear fruits, it's time to try out something new.

Chances are you'll succeed if you shift from your current weight loss invention to a better one. There is a wide variety of things you may want to change to achieve the results you've been waiting for several months or years. For example, you should consider doing something about the foods you eat, the types of exercises you do, and your current lifestyle habits.

Some of the weight loss regiments you'll come across will promise to solve your problem regardless of what you do, what you eat, and bodily functions. Well, you should be very careful because there is no single weight loss program that will work for everyone. The best approach is to use an individualized regimen based on things like your body weight, the foods you eat, metabolic rate, and the amount of calories in your body. These things are very important when developing a personalized weight loss program because they usually affect different people in different ways. For example, someone may eat certain foods and end up losing weight, but someone else might get different results after eating the same foods.

A personalized weight loss program is what you need to achieve the best results if you really want to lose weight. You need to make a smart decision, which is only possible if you know what your body needs. It is important to find out what your body needs with regard to diet, lifestyle habits, and exercise. Once you've discovered what is most likely to work for you, the next step is to start the weight loss process. Remember to motivate yourself so you can work hard to achieve your goal. With a clear understanding of what you have to do and the necessary motivation, you'll be able to lose the extra weight, have a healthier body, and get a well-sculpted body by the end of the weight loss process.

So far, you are aware of the fact that weight loss is not an easy job. You have to accept and keep this fact in mind before you start the journey. It's not one of the things you can do and expect to get the results you wanted by the end of the day. As mentioned earlier, weight loss is a process and every process includes steps that must be followed to get the best results. You need to follow each step of the process and exercise patience all the time because it may take several weeks or months before you lose a few pounds.

During the weight loss process, you have to make some adjustments for things to work properly. This includes making significant dietary changes, changing the way you exercise, getting rid of certain lifestyle habits, and adopting new lifestyle habits. Certainly, things won't be easy so you have to train yourself because there are other things to do in addition to following your weight loss program. For instance, you have to do the usual home-related tasks that could interfere with your weight loss plan. Your weight loss program may also make it difficult to follow your usual daily routine. Training for the process is essential to avoid unnecessary inconveniences.

Once you decide to embark on the weight loss journey, one of the major challenges you can expect is to make the first step. Every journey starts with a single step and you might come across some hurdles even when making the first step as you attempt to lose some pounds. Some of the obstacles you'll encounter exist even before you start the journey, so it might take some time before you adjust. The truth is that you have to be ready to adapt because no one will do the hard work for you.

You need to trust yourself and believe that everything is possible regardless of the challenges you are about to face. No challenge is impossible to overcome if you are strong-minded and ready to lose weight for a healthier body. Don't mind the challenges because you'll have something to smile about after the seemingly endless journey.

One of the most important things for any person who wishes to lose weight is to be ready for anything. However, you don't want to be deceived by weight loss regimen scams that promise everything. The best thing about this eBook is that it does not talk about deceptive workout plans, dieting programs, and costly clinical procedures that will produce no results or make you regret your decision. You are definitely looking for an effective weight loss regimen that will give you the results you need. Luckily, this book only focuses on real weight loss methods that will help you lose weight the correct way without causing complications.

You've made the right decision to read this book because the methods proposed here are safe. They are reliable weight loss methods that are effective in helping people achieve their weight loss goals. Read on if you want to be smart and make wise decisions regarding your weight loss plan.

If you've come this far, there's no doubt that you are ready to lose some pounds. We've mentioned food and diet several times and would like to take the discussion to the next level. Proceed to the next chapter to learn more about the types of foods your body needs as you begin your weight loss journey.

CHAPTER 2:

The Right Weight Loss Diet

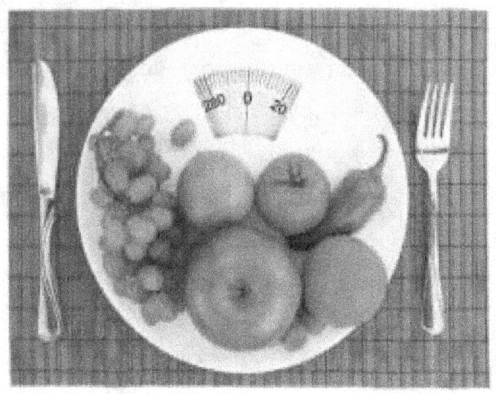

The food you eat every day is one of the key factors to keep in mind once you decide to start your weight loss journey. To some extent, the right food for you will be determined by the type of body you wish to have by the end of your weight loss journey. For example, if you want a slender body shape, you should look for and consume foods that will make you look thin. You can't expect to get a slender body if you choose to eat foods that will obviously make you fat.

One of the things you need to do in order to lose excess pounds in your body is to control the amount of calories you consume. It will be difficult to succeed in losing weight if you keep consuming more calories every day. Your body needs to get rid of the unwanted calories for you to stand a chance of losing weight. The amount of calories consumed should be less than the amount lost for your weight loss plan to work. In addition to controlling your calorie intake, it's important to pay attention to minerals and vitamins. You have to consume the correct amounts of these elements for your body to function properly.

Overall, you need to pay attention to everything you eat, and this brings us to our discussion about the right diet for individuals who want to lose weight. The right diet must contain the correct amounts of different components including calories, vitamins, proteins, fats, and minerals. Additionally, your diet must blend with your workout regimen well for you to achieve the best results. You'll certainly have a hard time if you expect to lose weight through dieting alone.

Your body muscles need to grow and gain strength, so you need to work out. However, you won't be able to work out and your muscles can't grow without food. Food provides the muscles with the nutrients and the energy they need. You can't expect to work out and come out victorious if your muscles are weak. As you can see, there is a significant relationship between diet and exercise when it comes to weight loss. You are required to maintain a balance between the two for your weight loss regimen to be successful. So, as you plan your exercise sessions, you must have a good source of nutrients. Avoid consuming foods with huge quantities of calories. This is important because one of the major steps you need to take is to lose those unwanted calories until you reach the recommended calorie count.

The Truth about Popular Fad Diets

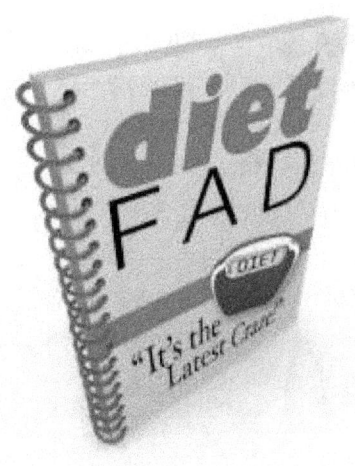

When looking for the appropriate weight loss diet, you need to know certain things first. You will come across many fad diets that promise to give you an instant solution, but they often end up giving you the wrong results even after using them for several weeks, months or years. A fad diet refers to a diet that purports to solve your weight gain problems with immediate effects. Usually, these diets are unhealthy and do not lead to weight loss. In fact, they may have devastating effects on your health and affect your overall wellbeing.

How to Identify a Fad Diet?

You should look for a number of characteristics to make sure you are not depending on a fad diet. As indicated earlier, fad diets claim to help people lose weight very quickly. Some of them will promise to help you lose several pounds in a week, which is often unrealistic. Fad diets also promise to help you lose weight without exercising. If you come across such diets or food products, stay away from them.

You can also identify a fad diet by checking the types of foods they contain because some of them lack essential nutrients. People who endorse fad diets or products also tend to use before-and-after pictures of someone who has apparently used their products and lost weight. You should be careful if you come across such diets. Finally, you should act with caution if you are asked to spend unreasonably high sums of money, especially if you are asked to pay for the diet or product in advance. Since fad diet plans are not as good as they claim to be, they are usually popular for a short time before they disappear.

Why You Should Say No to Fad Diets?

Fad diets do not perform miracles when it comes to weight loss. You have to avoid these diets at all costs because they will never give you the results you need. The first reason to avoid these foods is the fact that they often lack the nutrients your body needs to stay healthy. If you consume them, you are most likely to deprive yourself of essential elements like fats and carbohydrates. Your body with lack the energy it needs to stay strong if your diet lacks foods with these nutrients. Fad diets also remove essential vitamins meaning that your chances of having an unhealthy body are high if you depend on these diets.

In some cases, fad diets may actually help you lose a few pounds. This may sound like good news if you've tried other methods and failed, but the truth is that you won't be able to maintain your new weight for a long time. A fad diet may work if it contains the foods your body needs to maintain a healthy weight, but you will only enjoy the results for a short time. You want to use a diet plan that works for you and produces results that will last for the longest time possible.

One of the worst things you want to avoid is the risk of gaining more weight instead of losing weight. The problem with fad diets is that they can make you gain more weight than before and increase the risk of developing health problems that are associated with weight gain. If you decide to limit the volume of food you consume on a daily basis, your metabolic rate will drop. However, if you start consuming a lot of food on a regular basis, your metabolic rate will go up. As a result, your appetite will intensify and reach levels it has never reached before. When this happens, you will start to gain extra pounds, which is unfortunate. You can't afford to gain weight during the weight loss process, so you should ward off fad diets.

Another reason to keep off fad diets is the feeling that comes after realizing that things didn't work as you expected. One thing you'll notice about fad diets is that they give you hope and make you feel secure before you start consuming them. Unfortunately, users usually end up feeling hopeless and even scared to try another weight loss method once their fad diets fail. If you happen to try out a fad diet and fail miserably, you will lose your self-esteem and confidence, and it's not easy to rise up again. Weight loss may be a challenging process but it should not make you suffer or end up frightened. You should be able to use your money on the foods you love without exposing yourself to unnecessary suffering. In fact, you can actually splurge occasionally without risking your life as long as you know what is right for you.

You are also likely to find yourself in uncomfortable situations if you choose to follow a restrictive fad diet plan. For instance, you will have difficulty dining out because your diet restricts you from eating certain foods. If you happen to go out with your friends or people you can't afford to reject their offer, then you'll find yourself in a weird situation like a stranded stranger who doesn't know where to go or what to do. You'll be frustrated if you eventually decide to break the rules just to avoid disappointing other people.

Fad diets usually give all kinds of good promises and guarantee to produce the results you want within a very short duration. It's not surprising to come across a commercial featuring someone who claims to have lost thirty pounds in two weeks. This is the kind of message many people who want to lose weight get to hear, but the bad news is that the promises made by fad diet advertisers are usually false. As we said earlier in the book, weight loss is a process that takes time before you get the desired results. You have to wait for several weeks or months before you see significant changes.

In sum, once you begin your weight loss journey, bear in mind that you'll encounter all types of success stories, ads, and people endorsing potentially harmful diets. Most of these diets will leave you disappointed because they won't help you achieve your goals. If you are not careful, they will make you suffer and even deprive you of your favorite meals. Nothing will make you feel more frustrated than a fad diet that promises to help you lose weight only to make you gain more pounds. It's the most useless outcome you can get after all the hard work. In the end, you'll hate yourself just because you chose to lose weight the wrong way.

Luckily, you have the opportunity to lose those extra pounds the right way if you do the things recommended in this book. Now that you are aware of the risks of fad diets, make sure you avoid them and follow the right path away from unhealthy foods. If you've tried such diets and failed to get good results, you can now lose weight the correct way without avoiding your favorite foods. You don't want to make yourself suffer for making bad decisions. The best strategy is to have a diet plan that will help you eat healthier foods. You may have to limit yourself, but you don't have to avoid the foods you love even if they are considered to be unhealthy.

The Healthy Weight Loss Diet

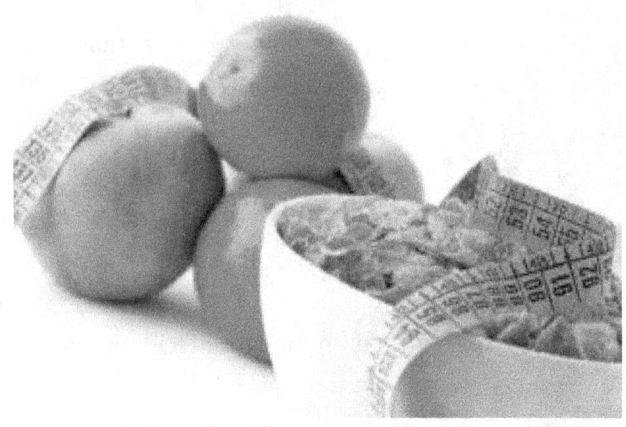

Now that you know the types of foods you have to avoid as you make the first step of your weight loss journey, let's talk about the healthy weight loss diet. You need a diet that will help you achieve your weight loss goals without harming your body. One of the things you should pay attention to during the weight loss process is the amount of calories in your diet. It's important to reduce the volume of calories for you to lose the excess body weight. Remember that eating fewer calories does not mean denying yourself food. It is possible to enjoy eating the foods you love on condition that you eat the right foods the right way.

Fiber-Rich Foods for Weight Loss

A healthy diet with the right elements is the first thing you need if you want to lose weight the right way. The most effective diets must include important components and the first one on the list is fiber. Fiber is basically a type of roughage found in different types of foods. It passes through the digestive system without being digested and plays a number of important roles. Fiber helps keep the digestive system healthy and clean, eases bowel movements, and helps the body get rid of harmful carcinogens and cholesterol.

The two types of fiber are soluble and insoluble fiber. As the name suggests, soluble fiber dissolves in water. It helps the body stay healthy by lowering blood sugar and cholesterol levels. On the other hand, insoluble fiber is the bulky fiber that does not dissolve in water. Your body needs it to prevent constipation. Generally, fiber-rich foods take a lot of space, stay longer in the digestive system, and make you full for longer durations. If you eat these foods, you'll feel relieved from hunger and end up consuming smaller amounts of calories. In the end, you'll be able to lose weight without depending on dangerous fad diets. Fortunately, it is easy to find fiber-rich foods that will help you lose some pounds in a healthy way. We'll now talk about healthy foods with large quantities of fiber for your weight loss diet.

Vegetables and Fruits

Vegetables and fruits are among the most important components of a healthy diet. For many years, people around the globe have known that a healthy diet must include vegetables and fruits. There are all kinds of vegetables and fruits to choose from depending on your preferences. They come in all colors and shapes, so it is easy to find a good choice. Vegetables and fruits have many health benefits to the human body and play a vital role in preventing a wide variety of health problems. They are rich in essential nutrients. No single vegetable or fruit contains all the necessary nutrients, so it is advisable to eat different varieties every day.

If you are looking forward to losing some weight, consider eating fiber-rich fruits like peaches, apples, and strawberries. Your weight loss diet should also include healthy salads with some green leafy vegetables. These will nourish your body with essential minerals and vitamins that will help you stay healthy. In addition, vegetables and fruits are a great option if you need to boost your appetite.

Whole Grains

We can't talk about fiber-rich foods without mentioning whole grains. Basically, whole grains are the seeds or grains of cereals or pseudocereals that contain the germ, the endosperm, and the bran. The germ is the inner layer that contains protein, minerals, and vitamins while the endosperm is the middle layer that contains large amounts of carbohydrates. The bran is the hard, outer layer that contains fiber, antioxidants and minerals. You need to avoid refined grains because they only retain the middle layer of the grain.

Whole grains are an important component of your weight loss diet because they provide your body with incredible amounts of fiber and carbohydrates. They are a great source of the energy needed to perform everyday tasks. The recommended fiber-rich whole grains for your diet include oatmeal, rice, bread, and pasta. One great thing about whole grains is that they are easy to use when preparing recipes. For example, you can easily prepare different types of recipes using pasta and always end up with a healthy dish that will help you achieve your weight loss objectives.

Beans

Beans also play a crucial role in the weight loss process. You need to include them in your diet because they are rich in fiber and proteins. They also contain decent amounts of phosphorus, potassium, magnesium, carbohydrates, folate, iron, vitamins, and calcium depending on the type you choose. In fact, many people who want to lose weight or work out consider beans to be an important element in their meals. It is easy to find beans for the perfect weight loss diet because they are available in all shapes and colors. Some of the best beans with significant amounts of fiber include peas, green peas, chickpeas and many more. They will not only help you lose some weight but also nourish your body with essential nutrients.

How to Prepare the Perfect Weight Loss Diet?

So far, we know that a good diet for anyone who wants to lose weight must include foods that are rich in fiber. These include different types of vegetables, fruits, whole grains, and beans. However, your diet must have the right amounts of each of these foods in order to achieve the best results. Of course, you'll need all of these foods, but you should mainly focus on vegetables and fruits to create the perfect weight loss diet.

Some of the health problems we face today are as a result of the things we do when it comes to diet. For instance, there are people who eat meals with large quantities of meat, which is not healthy at all. Interestingly, most of us eat meals with 80% meat content on a regular basis. If you've been eating meals with huge amounts of beef, pork or chicken, you should do something before it's too late. Some of the people who eat such meals tend to measure portions and count calories, which means they may not enjoy eating their food. You can avoid such problems by making changes to your diet. Make sure you include vegetables and fruits as the key components in your meals and you won't need to worry about calories.

You already know that it is important to regulate the amounts of calories you consume if you want your weight loss plan to succeed. If you include vegetables and fruits in your weight loss diet play, you'll always feel safe because calories will be the least of your worries. Vegetables and fruits will help you prepare a heavy and healthy meal. After some weeks or months, you'll see what these two can do if you consume the correct quantities.

We've already learned that foods that are rich in fiber will help you satiate your hunger and make you feel relieved within a very short time. Vegetables and fruits will make you feel satisfied almost immediately and you can stay for long periods without the urge to eat again. Of course, you can't just wake up and start eating vegetables and fruits without a good plan. You want to make the most of the nutrients contained in vegetables and fruits. Let's see how you can eat vegetables and fruits to get the best results.

1. *Eat Steamed or Raw Vegetables*

When it comes to vegetables in weight loss diets, it's important to know how they should be prepared to maximize the benefits. It is always advisable to eat steamed or raw vegetables because they contain more nutrients than thoroughly cooked vegetables. When in their natural form, vegetables provide your body with large quantities of nutrients. In contrast, cooked vegetables have their nutrients drained and thus lack the nutrients your body needs to stay healthy.

Each type of vegetable has its own taste and you can make it taste better by adding various ingredients. For instance, you could add some spices, herbs or a small amount of olive oil. Cheese is also a great option if you wish to improve the flavor.

2. Add Some Cheese and Nuts to Salads

You can also create the perfect diet by adding some cheese or nuts to salads. However, you should be careful when adding any of the two because you are only required to consume them in small quantities. Your main goal is to lose a few or several pounds, so you don't want to eat foods with large quantities of fat. Both cheese and nuts are known to contain fats, so you should make sure you only add small amounts to your weight loss diet. The best thing to do is to add low-fat salad dressings to your diet to add flavor without increasing calorie levels. Some of the best options include low-fat cheese and olive oil vinaigrette.

3. Eat More Fruits and Fewer Cereals during Breakfast

Nowadays, different types of cereals have become an important part of our everyday breakfast. Cereals are good, but you should avoid eating them in huge quantities. The best breakfast for any person who wishes to lose some pounds should contain less cereal and more fruits. Some of the recommended fruits to eat during breakfast include bananas, blueberries, and strawberries. With the right combination of cereals and fruits, you will enjoy your usual cereals and also eat a meal with fewer calories. It will be tasty and probably taste better than what you've been eating.

4. *Replace Cheese and Meat with Healthier Vegetables*

One of the best things to do when you begin your weight loss journey is to reduce the amount of cheese and meat in your meals. Both foods contain some fat, which you should avoid because you can't risk getting fat in the process of losing weight. Try to replace some of the cheese or meat with healthier vegetables.

There are different types of vegetables to choose from including tomatoes, cucumber, lettuce and many more. These vegetables will help you prepare a healthy meal with smaller amounts of calories. You should consider using them in quick meals. They provide the body with essential nutrients, give you energy, and help you lose some pounds at the same time.

5. *Avoid Junk Foods*

Jung foods generally refer to processed foods with low nutritional value. If you need something to relieve your hunger quickly, stay away from foods like fried fast foods, cookies, salted snacks, and sugary carbonated drinks. The problem with junk foods is that they usually don't make you feel full. As a result, you are likely to eat more food. Additionally, people tend to replace other healthy foods with junk foods. Instead of drinking healthy beverages like fruit juice and green tea, some people drink a lot of soda, which is unhealthy. You should avoid junk foods and eat some carrots, healthy dips, and corn. Hummus is an excellent choice if you are interested in dips.

6. *Include Vegetables in Your Main Course Recipes*

When it comes to main courses, you want to ensure that your recipes contain some vegetables. If you include vegetables in your main course recipes, you'll be able to prepare more rewarding dishes, add color to your meals, make your meals taste more delicious than before, and enjoy meals packed with nutritious components. Even if you are a fan of stir-fried meals, pasta and noodles, you can make them more nutritious and healthier by adding some vegetables.

7. *Start Meals with Appetizers*

Another important thing to keep in mind is to eat something to stimulate your appetite before you eat your meals. Some popular appetizers include healthy soup and salads. If you start your meals with appetizers, you'll be able to relieve your hunger before you even start the main meal. This is a great strategy because you need to eat less if you want to lose some weight. It helps you avoid consuming huge volumes of foods that might worsen the situation by making your body gain weight. You don't want this to happen, so make sure you start all meals with an appetizer.

How to Work with Your Favorite Foods in Your Diet?

People who want to lose weight usually have to deal with the pressure to stay away from their favorite foods. When dieting for the sake of losing weight, people are told they can't enjoy their comfort foods, which is a big misconception. The truth is that it is possible to eat your comfort foods even if you are on a weight loss diet. Of course, you may be required to avoid some of the foods you eat if they are deemed unhealthy for someone who is trying to lose weight However, it does not mean that you can't eat them.

Who said it's wrong to have a piece of chocolate occasionally? Even though you are trying to stay healthy by avoiding unhealthy foods including your favorites, you can still have a chocolate bar because it won't have a significant impact on your diet. However, you must make sure that the meals you eat contain the correct quantities of vegetables, fruits, and whole grains as advised earlier in this book. If you are confident that your meals have the recommended foods, you can still eat your favorite foods by following a number of steps. We'll now talk about how to work with your favorite foods in your diet.

1. Have Treats at Specific Times

If you love treats and you still want to have some, feel free to eat them even when on a weight loss diet. However, you should not eat your favorite snacks every time you feel like eating. The best way to eat them if you really want to lose weight is to have a proper schedule. For example, you may decide to have them in the form of a reward after doing something useful such as studying. You may also have a small chocolate bar after your lunchtime meal or have a piece of cake when you go out on Saturdays. A schedule for eating treats will help you work with snacks without getting obsessed with your favorite treats.

2. Have Treats with Healthy Foods

When on a healthy weight loss diet, you want to minimize the effects of potentially unhealthy treats as much as possible. One way to do this is to eat your treats with healthy foods. This is a great option because you'll not only have your treats but also have a meal packed with nutrients. In addition, the meal will help to satiate your hunger. So, if you want to have some ice cream, you can do it as long as you do things the right way. You only need to eat your ice cream with foods that contain low amounts of calorie. Since you are combining foods with less calorie count with your favorite treats, you are confident that you won't gain weight. Make sure you moderate your treats to avoid unwanted results.

3. Use Your Senses

In addition to having foods with nutritional value, good meals look great, taste good, and have a nice aroma. For that reason, you need to indulge your nose, eyes, taste buds, and ears. If you want to eat some treats, it is important to focus on how the meal looks and the aroma. A great aroma will definitely help boost your appetite and the good news is that you can easily create a scented environment for your meal. For instance, you can choose to purchase scented candles to create an aromatic ambience. Try it and you'll be more than happy to indulge your nose.

4. Make Your Treats Healthier

If you know you are going to eat a lot of treats, then you should make them healthier because you want to eliminate the risk of gaining weight. There are different ways to make your snacks healthier including using small quantities of fat, reducing the amount of sugar, and using healthier ingredients. For example, you can replace your chocolate cake with a carrot or banana cake that does not contain sugar.

If you choose healthier ingredients, you'll be able to eat your favorite treats and realize your weight loss goals without unnecessary struggles. Sugar-free treats still taste good, so feel free to try them out and share with your friends and family members.

This chapter has helped you understand the key elements of a healthy diet for people who want to lose weight. Without a doubt, diet is a very important aspect of the weight loss process. When creating your weight loss regimen, you must consider things like calorie count and fats. The human body gains calories depending on the types of foods we eat, so it is important to focus on the ingredients we use to prepare meals. The perfect weight loss meal is packed with essential nutrients with nutritional benefits to the body. It provides the body with the energy it needs to get things done every day.

Exercise plays an important role in helping overweight or obese people lose weight. Physical activity will help you lose the extra fat in your body, but it is useless if you adopt unhealthy eating habits. Even if you have the best workout plan on earth, you must pay attention to the types of foods you eat, eating time, and the quantity of food you consume every day. It is difficult to achieve your goals if you fail to create a perfect balance when it comes to the different types of foods you need to include in your diet. You should have a steady diet program and remember that you don't have to deny yourself your favorite treats. Feel free to eat your conform foods even when on a weight loss diet provided you do it the right way.

All in all, you need a diet with healthy foods to lose weight the correct way. Now that we've mentioned exercise, read the next chapter to learn more about the best exercises for your weight loss regimen.

CHAPTER 3:

The Best Exercises for Weight Loss

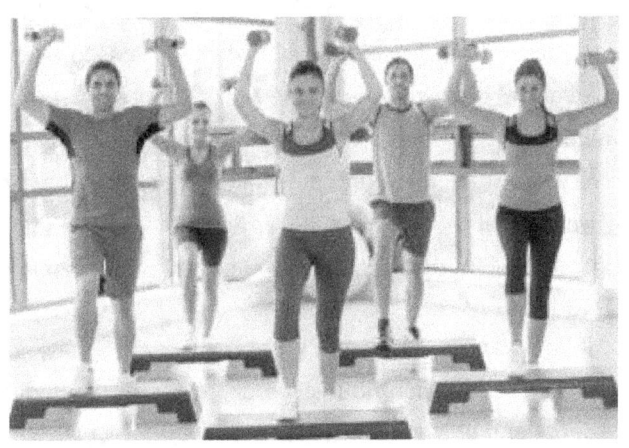

We now know that diet is a key aspect of an effective weight loss regimen mainly because of the role it plays in determining your calorie intake. Once you come up with a diet with the right types of healthy foods, the next step is to engage in some form of physical activity. Exercises are important because they will help you lose weight by getting rid of the extra fat that has accumulated in your body. Since you already know the types of foods you need to include in your weight loss diet, it's time to talk about exercises and workouts that will help you lose the excess pounds the right way. People who want to lose weight have been using weight loss exercises and workouts for many years, so it's nothing new.

Some of the weight loss regimens you'll come across include different types of exercises that help you lose the excess fat in various parts of the body such as around the arms, the stomach, and the thighs. When it comes to weight loss diet, we've learnt that fad diets will promise to produce the desired results without exercising. Such diets will only leave you disappointed and may have devastating impacts on your health. They are often deceptive. The most effective weight loss program combines diet and exercises.

So, if you want to lose some weight the healthy way, you must eat foods that nourish your body with essential nutrients and engage in physical activity. Your weight loss program should focus on eating the right foods and doing enough exercises so as to achieve the best results. Even if your diet contains the healthiest foods anyone can find on the market today, it will be of no use if you still have an inactive lifestyle. For example, if you eat healthy foods and still sit on your couch or sit in the office the whole day, chances are you won't get the results you expect unless you do some physical exercises.

A diet with healthy foods provides your body with the nutrients you require to stay healthy and generate energy every day. Exercises will improve your muscle tones in addition to helping you lose the unwanted fat. Eventually, you'll lose the excess weight in different parts of the body and achieve your desired body shape. The key point here is that you won't be able to lose weight by just eating a diet with healthy foods. You must combine diet with exercises to get great results. In fact, some studies have revealed that the best way to maintain the ideal body weight is through physical activity.

How to Exercise?

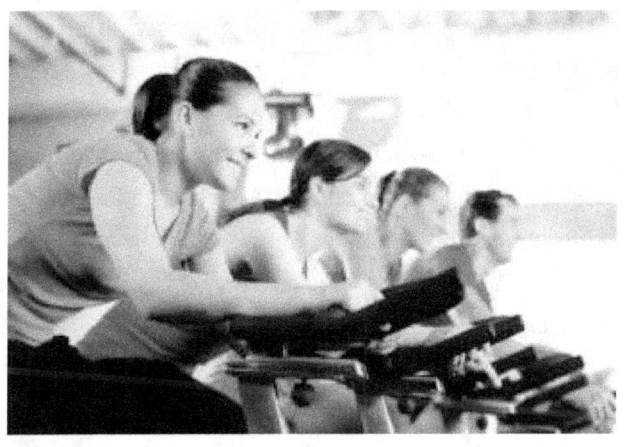

You definitely want to know how often and for how much you need to exercise in order to get the best results during the weight loss process. It is important for everyone who wants to lose some pounds to know how much they need to exercise because you don't want to mess things up by doing things the wrong way. Bodybuilders may advise you to do vigorous exercises every day. Other people will tell you to do shorter exercises occasionally.

With this kind of information, you may have trouble making the right decision when it comes to weight loss exercises. To be honest, there's no specific way to exercise because it depends on various factors that differ from one person to another. Your exercise needs may be different from another person's needs.

Although you want to do everything possible to get rid of the excess fat, it does not necessarily mean that you must exercise on a regular basis. You don't need to engage in physical activity every day in order to lose those extra pounds. The most important thing is to exercise a number of times per week. For example, you can decide to exercise four or five times every week and get good results by the end of your weight loss journey. People who believe that overweight persons should exercise every day will probably disagree with this type of exercise plan. However, you should give your body enough time to heal, so there's nothing wrong with getting exercise four or five times every week.

Any form of physical activity can damage your muscles and that's why it is important to give your body some time to rest. If you are exercising four to five days a week, you have 2 to 3 days to rest. During this period, your body will heal and prepare itself for the following week's exercise. Professional athletes usually work out on a regular basis, but they also give themselves some time to eat, relax, and gain more energy for the next exercise. The body gets a chance to recover during the rest period. When you start your exercises, make sure you give your body a chance to rest and eat the foods recommended in the previous chapter to give your muscles the required energy. Two rest days will be enough.

As mentioned earlier in this chapter, several factors will determine how much exercise you need in order to lose weight. One of these factors is your stamina, which refers to the ability to endure or stay strong during workouts. When developing your workout plan, you need to keep in mind what your body can handle before you engage in intense exercises that demand high levels of endurance. Start with a simple exercise that your body can withstand and gradually introduce more demanding exercises.

It is wrong to start things off with intense exercises if you haven't done it before because the chances of harming your body are extremely high. If you start with intense exercises, you will get tired quickly before you even reach your target for that day. You'll eventually get nothing from your workout plan if you continue doing exercises the wrong way. The best strategy is to begin with simple exercises that will not expose your body to too much stress or unhealthy physical activity before you move to energy-intensive exercises. You don't want to end up hurting yourself in the process.

Based on our previous discussion, you'll realize that the two most important factors you need to pay attention to when exercising are duration and intensity. Your workout regimen should allow you to start with shorter exercises that do not require a lot of energy. For example, you can choose to start with stretches that last for 15 minutes and work your way up by gradually adding more minutes. After doing the stretches, you can start some jogging exercises that last for about 10 minutes. Once your body gets used to the exercise, feel free to move to 15 to 30-minute jogging exercises.

Make sure you don't change things abruptly because you want to work on your stamina one step at a time. If you change the duration of each exercise quickly, you should also expect to get exhausted quickly. Your body needs to get used to one type of physical activity before you do intense exercises such as sprinting and lifting weights. Generally, the best way to exercise is to start with shorter exercises and gradually introduce intense exercises until your body is able to do engage in more intense physical activities.

The Right Weight Loss Exercises

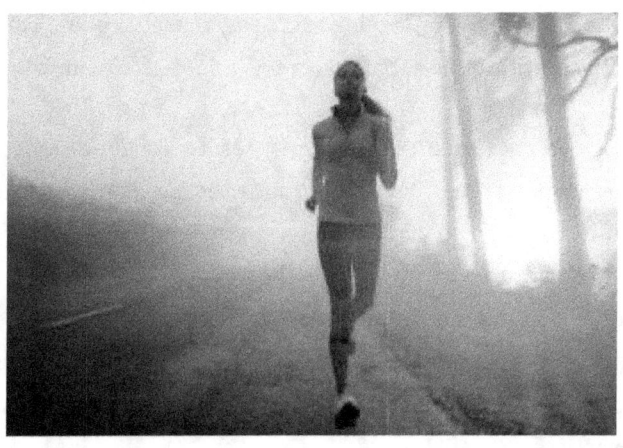

People who wish to shave off some pounds usually have difficulty choosing from the wide variety of exercises that are recommended for weight loss. If you are unable to figure out the types of exercise you need to do to burn the unwanted fats, we've done research on your behalf and identified the right weight loss exercises for you. We've found various options including jogging, weight lifting, yoga, swimming, and cycling. You'll definitely find the right exercise for you from the list. Let's talk about these exercises in detail.

Jogging

If you've exercised or watched other people do exercises, you've probably noticed that jogging is a popular exercise in many exercise regiments. It's a great choice to start with because it helps improve your stamina. Jogging does not require a lot of movement, so you won't get tired quickly. When starting your jogging exercises, make sure you start with short distances that take a few minutes to complete.

Once you get used to short distances, try longer distances and increase the intensity of your exercise. Remember to do it gradually to avoid damaging your muscles. You also don't want to hurt your feet in the process, so find yourself some nice shoes once you start jogging for longer distances. If you reach a point where your body gets used to intense jogging exercising, it's time to shift to more intense exercises.

Weight Lifting

The second exercise on our list of weight loss exercises is weight lifting. This type of exercise has been around for many years and is definitely here to stay. It is an important part of your weight loss regiment because it plays a vital role in helping the body burn those extra calories. In fact, weight lifting helps the body burn calories almost instantly. However, you need to know that it can harm your body if you do it the wrong way. You are at a greater risk of harming yourself if you are doing it for the first time.

As a beginner, it's advisable to look for an experienced person to help you. If possible, visit a gym and find a professional trainer who will ensure you don't harm your body in the process. The trainer will also teach you how to use the various equipment you'll be using every time you visit the gym to exercise.

Yoga

Yoga is another effective exercise if you want to take things slowly. It is a great option every time you feel like stretching your body. There are different types of yoga positions that will help your body become more flexible. If you watch people doing yoga, you might think it's a simple exercise. However, the truth is that yoga is a challenging exercise that will make you sweat and even make your joints ache. One of the benefits of doing yoga is that you can work out alone at home without using special equipment. You can do it on your mat as long as you are comfortable. If you like working out at home, then do some yoga.

Swimming

If you want to lose weight and you love swimming, you can get rid of excess body fat by doing what you love. However, you don't have to be an experienced swimmer to go swimming. Once you get into the water, there are different ways to have fun including moving around. As you move around, you'll be using your muscles to move your joints and the water will keep you comfortable by making your body float. If you swim regularly, your joints will eventually achieve maximum mobility. Whether you love swimming in pools or the ocean and you want to lose weight, make sure you get into the pool or visit the beach from time to time.

Bicycle Riding

You can also lose weight by cycling along the road. Bicycle riding is an exciting activity because you can ride while going to work or school. If possible, find yourself a good bicycle and ride around town whenever you get a chance. You will enjoy the ride and get rid of some weight in the process. Cycling is a great choice if you already own a bicycle. Take advantage of it if you enjoy cycling.

In this chapter, we've learnt that your weight loss regimen cannot be effective without some form of exercise. You need to eat the right foods and choose the right exercises in order to lose weight in a healthy way. The key factors to consider when exercising include the duration and intensity of the exercise. Your main objective is to use safe methods that will help you lose weight the right way, so you should avoid fad diets. In addition, you need to ignore all advertisements that promise to help you lose weight without involving a good exercise plan.

Any weight loss regimen without exercise is a misleading plan for lazy people who are not ready to do the hard work. Without exercise, you'll end up wasting your time and money. If you are really determined to lose some pounds, stop sitting on your couch and get up to do some exercise.

Look for some nice sneakers and head to the gym. Lift weights, do some yoga exercises, swim, and ride your bicycle to get every muscle working. Exercise the right way and you'll lose weight the right way.

Conclusion

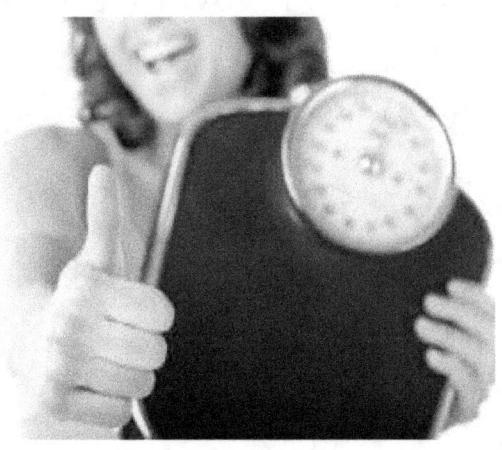

The weight loss journey is often described as difficult, worthless, vague, and impossible. We have to acknowledge that weight loss is a challenging task that requires hard work, time, and money. It's not easy to achieve good results unless you are persistent and patient. You must be prepared to work hard and face all the challenges in order to get what you want.

Today, there are many overweight and obese people who want to lose weight and some have failed because they don't know the correct way to lose weight. There are so many fad diets making it difficult for people to find an effective weight loss method.

Luckily, we've discussed the best weight loss methods in this book. The most important components of an effective weight loss regimen include a diet with healthy foods and exercise. The best way to lose the excess fat in your body is to make sure your diet plan works well with your exercise plan. Your diet should contain a wide variety of healthy foods, especially fruits and vegetables. Also, you should do the exercises recommended in this book to lose weight the right way without developing complications.

In addition to eating the right food and doing the right exercises, it is important to have the right attitude towards losing weight. The only person who can motivate you to keep pushing is you, so self-drive is a key factor. Don't wait for other people to motivate you because some of them will discourage you.

Obviously, you are not going to get what you want immediately. Losing weight the healthy way requires commitment and determination because you are going to face one challenge after another. Once you start the journey, you should work hard to complete it and prepare to face all the challenges. By the end of the journey, you'll be happy with yourself for not giving up along the way. Apart from losing some weight, you'll enjoy other benefits including improved self-confidence and opportunities that can only come if you have the right body weight. Generally, weight loss has significant impacts on your overall wellbeing.

Now that you know the right way to lose weight, there's no need to keep waiting. This book has provided you with every piece of information you needed to know about the correct way to lose weight. Would you like to start the process? Well, don't wait for tomorrow, next week, next month, or next year. The time is NOW! All you need to do is to start out with the correct diet, do the right exercises, and adopt healthier lifestyle habits. It's quite a journey, but it can only start if you make the first step

.

Paolo Jose De Luna

www.ingramcontent.com/pod-product-compliance
Lightning Source LLC
Chambersburg PA
CBHW071126280526
45787CB00003B/1187